TABLE OF CONTENTS

Introduction

Hello and welcome to our brief introductory guide on basic stretching exercises designed to keep seniors healthy & limber.

Your body will be going through a lot of changes as you get older. Your hair becomes gray or white, your skin becomes wrinkled, and your body becomes rigid when you undergo joint, muscle, and bone problems. We have believed for several years that working up the joints and relaxing the muscles is a normal part of aging, but recent work indicates otherwise.

Research has now found that at least half of the changes undergone by elderly people with respect to their joints, muscles, and bones are a direct result of lack of exercise.

However, when less than 10 percent of people over the age of 50 do not get enough exercise to at least maintain their health, it is no wonder that so many people have accepted their destinies as normal.

Bone and Muscle Problems in the Aging Body

Bones in a joint do not touch one another directly. Cartilage that line your joints (articular cartilage), synovial membranes around the joint and a lubricating fluid within your joints (synovial fluid) cushion them. The joint movement is stiffer and less flexible as you age as the volume of lubricating fluid within the joints reduces and the cartilage is thinner. Likewise, ligaments tend to shorten and lose strength , making joints feel rigid.

Some of such age-related joint changes are due to lack of exercise. Joint motion, and the related movement 'pain,' helps to keep the fluid flowing. Inactivity causes the cartilage to shorten which stiffen, which limits joint mobility.

Muscle Changes

As we age, our muscles experience a lot of changes that contribute to the above problems. Our muscle fibers are becoming smaller and we have less of them, and changes in the nervous system result in less muscle tone and a decreased muscle contracting capacity. Missing muscle tissue is regenerated more gradually than before and the tissue that replaces it is robust and fibrous, too.

Bone Changes

We don't always think of bones as living tissue, but they are entirely and they often experience transition as we age. Our bones start losing more calcium and other essential minerals because of the hormonal changes that arise as we age. Women are especially vulnerable to menopause but the bone loss that occurs with age affects even men.

Joint Changes

The movement of our joints is the result of contraction of the ligament, the flow of synovial fluid covering the joints, and layers of cartilage preventing bones from coming into direct contact with one another. However, in the aging body, ligaments may become thinner and less flexible, there is less synovial fluid to lubricate joints, and thin to cartilage. It all causes the joints to stiffen.

How This Guide Can Help You

A large number of such age-related disorders can be reversed by routine exercise and stretching exercises, or avoided. This course focuses primarily on how to use stretching as a way of maintaining limberness and flexibility no matter how old you are. The fact is, getting to start doing something for your body is never too late.

Upon completion of this guide, you will have all the resources you need to keep your body in the best possible condition to enjoy your golden years

Chapter 1 – An Overview Of Stretching The Aging Body And Basic Anatomy

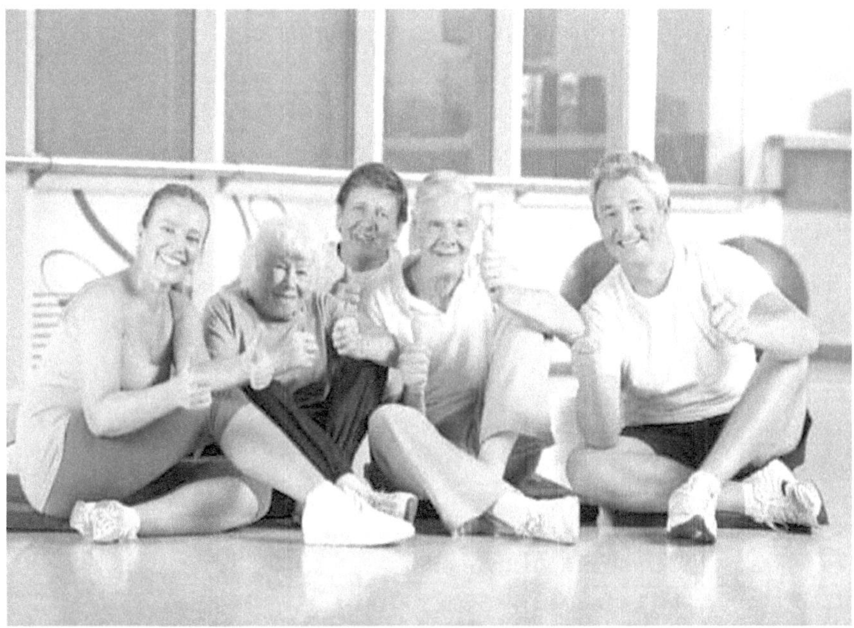

The primary objective of stretching the aging body is to prevent the disuse of muscles and joints from becoming stiff. Through relaxing your muscles frequently, and flexing your joints, you can help avoid many of the age-related problems affecting an aging body's joints, muscles, and bones. We're going to go through the main muscle groups and joints in this section of the guide which are most necessary to keep limber.

The 11 Major Muscle Groups

There are 11 major muscle groups you would like to make sure you use regularly and keep stretched out. If you do strength training workouts as well, these are the same muscle groups that you're going to work out with.

Forearms-There are many muscles in your lower arm that are particularly critical for raising and holding objects.

Biceps-A large muscle located in each of your upper arms that lets your forearms lift stuff.

Triceps-These are the other 2 muscles in the upper body. They help in stretching your body and bending your elbow.

Shoulders – There are a variety of muscles on your neck, back, and side that make up the shoulders that are responsible for raising your body.

Trapezius – These are the muscles in your upper back, also referred to as traps, that help move your spine, head, and shoulder blade.

Chest – This group of muscles covering your ribcage is responsible for assisting with arm movement and respiration.

Abdominals – This essential muscle group located in your abdomen helps breathe and protect your spine. They are often referred to as abs or the muscles of your core.

Back – The back muscles, one of the largest muscle classes, help protect the spine and are a part of hip motion.

Quadriceps-These are the four muscles located at the front of the thigh and are a vital part of the movement of the legs as they help control the movement of the hip and knee.

Hamstrings – The muscle group that makes up the back of the thigh and also assists with the hip and knee movement.

Calves-The muscles in your lower leg help you move your knee and bend your ankle.

The 7 Major Joints

Although you have a variety of smaller joints in your fingers and toes, there are seven big joints in the rest of your body that we must cover-up. Each joint consists of a combination of muscles providing the movement, ligaments, and tendons connecting bones and muscles, and bones.

Spine – Your spine helps protect the upper body and hold the nerves that connect through every device. It is composed of multiple individual vertebrae.

Shoulder-largely responsible for the motions of the entire neck.

Elbow – It helps with the lifting in the center of your head.

Wrist – Composed of many parts, the wrist is an integral part of hand movement.

Hip – Another ball-and-socket joint, this one is responsible for moving the entire body.

Knee-This joint on your leg helps you walk.

Ankle – Another joint, which has many sections, your ankle, can support your legs and help you walk.

In the next part, we will learn more about why stretching these muscle groups will support the aging body shell

Chapter 2 – Why Stretching is Beneficial to the Aging Body

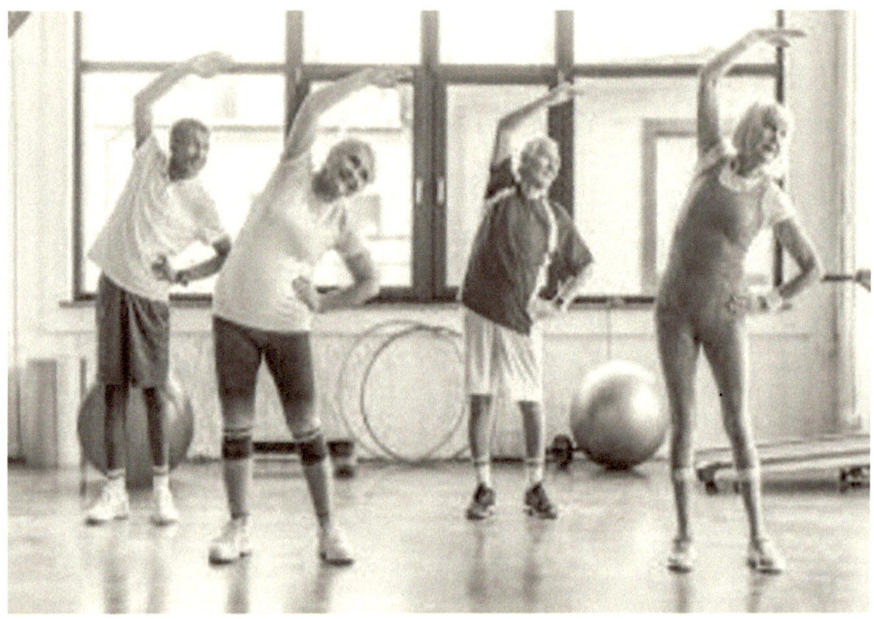

As we discussed earlier, there are a number of problems we face with our joints, muscles, and bones as our body ages. Luckily, we can do something about it and that is stretching. Stretching along with other physical activities can help prevent or even reverse many of the issues we talked about earlier.

Muscles and Stretching

They can become rigid if you don't use your muscles enough which leads to painful movements. You will prevent the muscles from becoming rigid by relaxing regularly and improve their elasticity. The more relaxed your muscles are, the less discomfort you'll feel when you're going about your day, and the more you can do it.

Another advantage of exercising your aging muscles frequently is that this will strengthen your balance. This is because when your muscles are relaxed regularly they will better respond to movements that help you stay balanced. It will not only allow you to be more comfortable as you do other workouts but will also help avoid falls that are especially dangerous to the aging body.

Bones and Stretching

Although stretching does not help to strengthen your bones, there are a variety of exercises to do, including walking, which you must do before each stretching session to warm your muscles up. If you have particular concerns about bone loss, you may want to make sure that you perform some basic exercises that will not only build bone mass but also relax exercises.

In addition, you can increase the range of motion in your joints by consistently relaxing, and encourage muscle strength that will allow you to do the exercises you need to do to make your bone health easier. When your muscles change and get stronger through exercise, your bones will recover the bone density that has been lost as you grow older.

Joints and Stretching

Stretching can help to keep the joints more flexible, which is important to aging bodies as joints tend to become more rigid with age and lose flexibility. You've got a wider range of motion, with more flexibility. This will help eliminate previously unpleasant movements from various forms of exercise along with daily activities.

The stretching of tendons in the joints offers another benefit. Tendons bind your muscles to your bones, and, if not in use, may become rigid and shorten over time. The best way to relax and lengthen the tendons is by periodically relaxing to get your joints working well again.

The other side of the joints are the ligaments which hold the bones. They should be solid and not very flexible, as they provide joint stability. However, with age, they can become too stiff, and stretching will help to get them back to where they are meant to be so instead of limiting your movements, relaxing your joints and allowing you to move freely.

Other Health Benefits to Stretching

Stretching has so many other health benefits, such as helping you relax, enhancing your posture, increasing stamina and energy levels, encouraging blood circulation, and raising cholesterol. Hold on reading through this course to learn more about stretching your aging body to improve your health.

Chapter 3 – Things to Consider Before Starting a Stretching Program

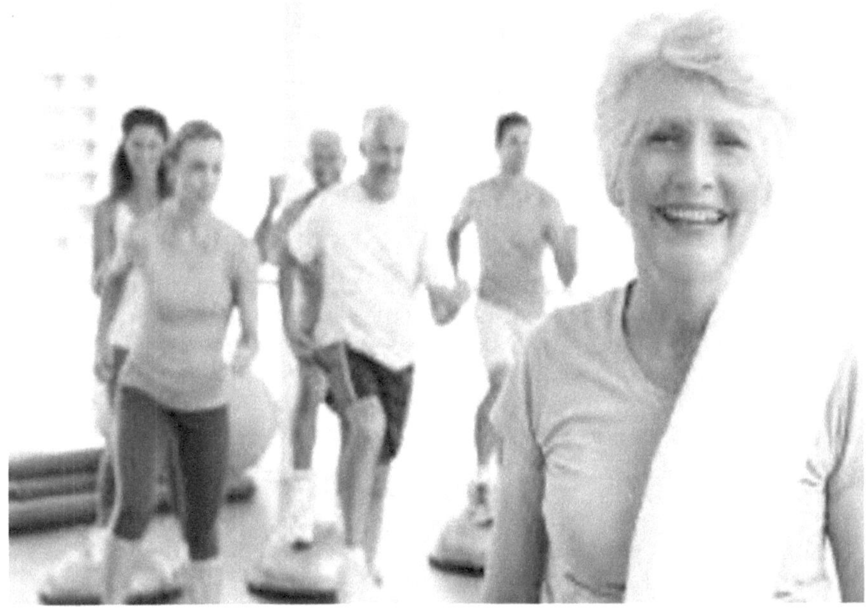

It's crucial that you do these things first before you start a stretching program. Even though starting stretching regularly may sound like an easy thing, if you aren't properly trained, you're at a far higher risk of injury. Preparation will also help you to know exactly what you are getting into, so you can stick to the program you choose.

Talk to Your Doctor

The most important thing to do before you initiate a stretching program is to talk to your doctor about your current health. He will be able to tell you which things you need to work on, and how much you need to stretch to improve your health safely. If you have problems with your bones or heart, you can start with medications or supplements as well.

Find a Trainer

If you're new to stretching, or your doctor suggests training with someone to concentrate on particular issues, then you'll need to find a trainer. You may be able to attend the classes or find someone via a nearby gym for general help with stretching.

If you do have physical disabilities, however, you may need to find a physical therapist to support.

Find a Location

It is best to find a place where you can do your stretching exercises with maximum ease and effectiveness. At home, at a gym or at your local community center, you can choose to do this. Since some stretches need some extra equipment, you will need to make sure that wherever you are, you have access to these. Many community centers will have small workout centers that are ideal for exercises and are generally much more affordable than gyms

Get Proper Clothing

Wearing the right clothes can help you stretch much easier, but it doesn't have to be anything too costly or fancy, so don't worry. You just want to wear clothes which do not in any way limit your movements. That can be tight-fitting clothes like spandex or yoga pants, but if that's more of your style, it can also be loose-fitting sweatpants.

Get Some Stretching Equipment

Without equipment, you can do many stretches but having some basic pieces of equipment will make some stretches easier and safer for your aging body. Stretch bands or resistance bands are great for facilitating and intensifying many stretches.

For different leg stretches, an incline board provides you with an angled surface, and a yoga mat is the best way to cushion your body when you do any stretches from the ground.

Also, there are a number of different machines specially designed for stretching. These are a great way to get started as they force you to do the stretch properly which helps to prevent injury and improve the stretch 's effectiveness.

Unfortunately, these are generally quite expensive, so if you're able to find a gym that has them, that's a better option.

Once you've got everything packed, the only thing left to do is to continue reading to learn more about stretching and start stretching every day.

Chapter 4 – Types Of Stretches & Timing

We 're going to go through the various types of stretches that are performed in this section of the course, and which form of stretching would be better for you and your aging body. We will also discuss why timing stretches are important, and how much time you should take for each stretch.

Ballistic Stretching

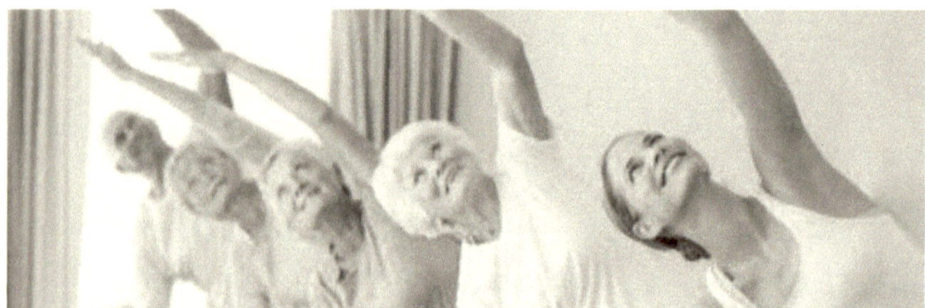

If you've ever seen someone jump when stretching, this is ballistic stretching. The idea is to push a joint beyond its normal range of motion using the momentum of your movement.

It is one form you can avoid at all costs because your muscles can sometimes get tighter or cause injury.

Active Stretching

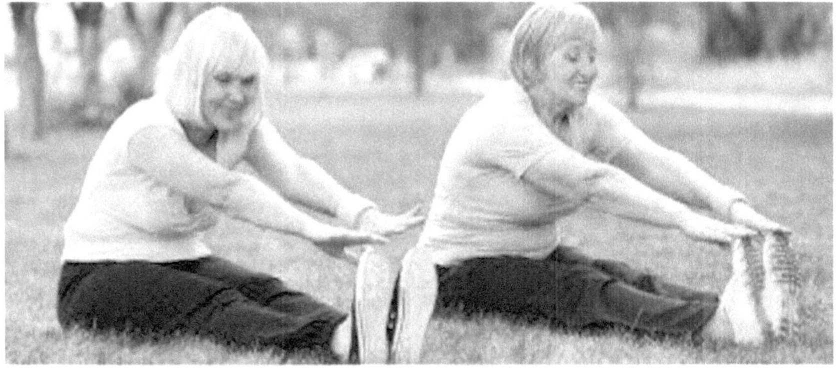

Also used in yoga, this includes holding the limb in place without any support from props or other limbs and allowing the stretch to be done only by the muscles inside that limb. This can be incredibly challenging which is why it is rarely kept at a time for more than 10 seconds, but it is also perfect for muscle building.

Passive stretching

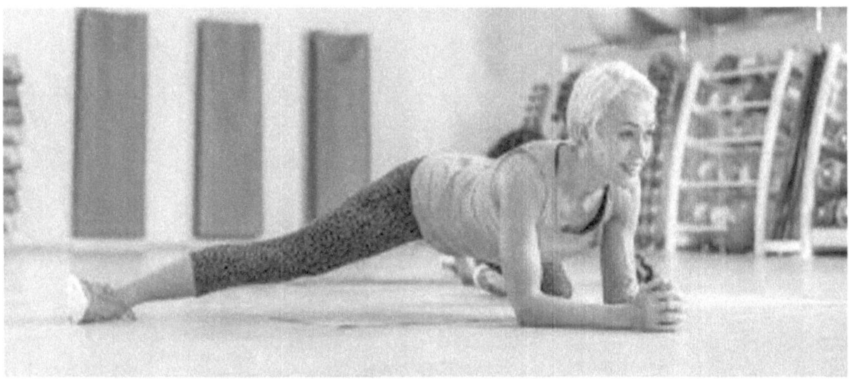

You assume and hold a position Like active stretching, passive stretching. Such stretches, however, are kept for a much longer period of time (1 minute or more) because they use props that allow you to hold the stretch. These are great for injuries because the muscles aren't working too hard.

Isometric Stretching

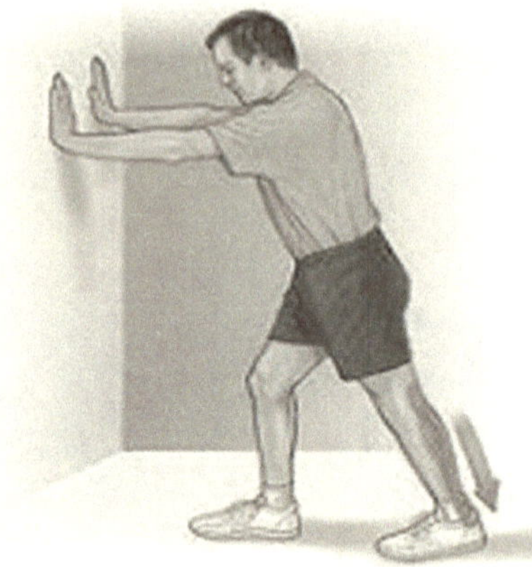

This kind of stretching involves pushing past the passive stretch using your own strength. You assume a position and then push against the prop (or in some cases your trainer) to create a deeper stretch on those muscles which is a great way to engage more muscle fibers than just passive stretching.

Dynamic stretching

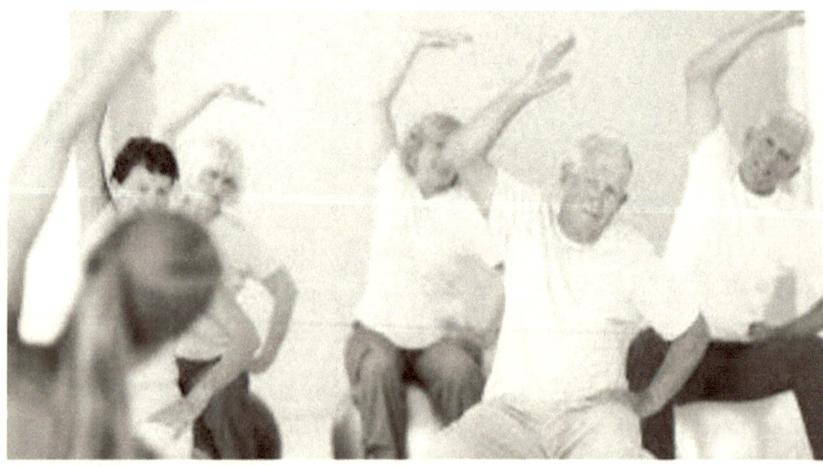

This is another form of stretching which involves motion but is safe and beneficial. You perform sets of specific leg and arm movements with dynamic stretching that allow your joints to gently and naturally extend beyond their previous limits, exercising them and flexing the muscles simultaneously.

PNF Stretching

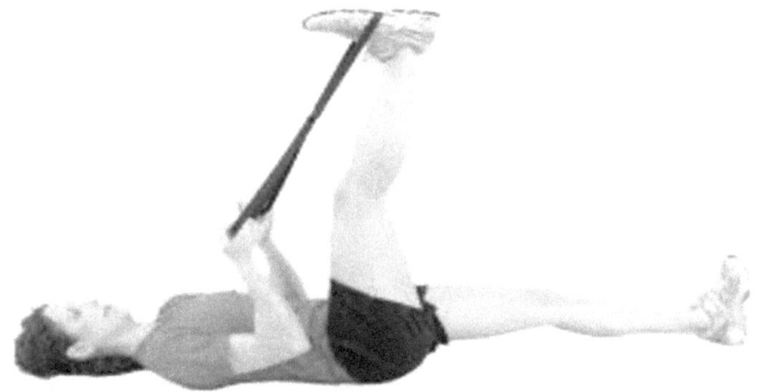

PNF stands for proprioceptive neuromuscular facilitation, and a combination of passive and isometric stretches is essentially used to deliver even better results than one of those techniques alone. This is the fastest way to improve flexibility through stretching, because of the combination of stretches.

Timing of stretches

As we have mentioned before, different streets are kept for various periods of time. As with active and dynamic stretches, this is often linked to stretch complexity, but stretch effectiveness is also a factor. While an active stretch will take just 10 seconds to be successful, performing a passive stretch for the same period of time will not produce any results.

Because most passive and isometric stretches require at least one minute for each of the major muscles, you'll need to make sure you 're giving yourself plenty of time for each stretching session. Allowing your muscles to stretch for at least one minute each allows them to stretch and maintain this position gradually, as long as they can affect that muscle for more than a few minutes after your session

Chapter 5 - Popular Stretch Training Programs & Their Effectiveness

There are two types of programs that are most common when it comes to stretch training: yoga, and Pilates. But before you sign up for the next class that will be offered in your city, we'll explore exactly what these stretch training programs are and help you decide how good they are for you and your aging body.

What's Yoga About?

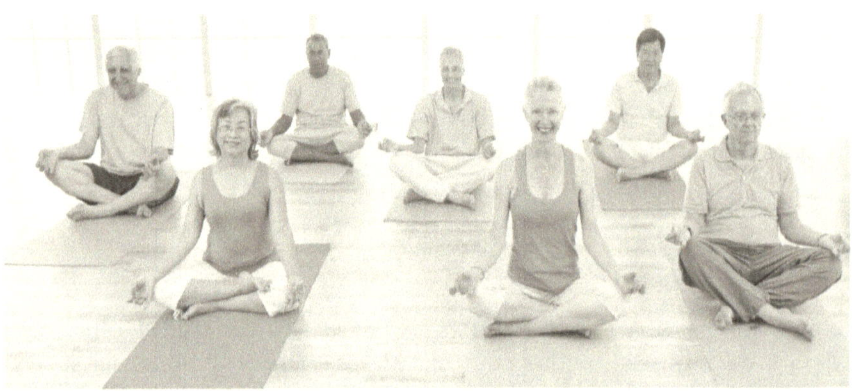

Yoga originated as a spiritual discipline developed by Hindus to combine control of breathing, meditation, and different poses of the body to create spiritual connections. You can also find many people who simply concentrate on the wellness benefits of yoga, using both active and passive stretches.

What are Yoga 's Advantages?

Some of the benefits of regularly practicing yoga include increased strength and endurance, enhanced blood flow, can be used as physical therapy for specific conditions, and relief from stress. Although there are definitely some difficult poses, an experienced coach can help you execute adapted variations of these poses or help you find poses that can give you the same stretch.

What are the Benefits of Yoga?

First of all, you can stop Bikram or Hot Yoga because there is evidence that this can be harmful to your safety. But beyond that, the biggest disadvantage to yoga is having an instructor who drives you too hard to hurt yourself while doing something you shouldn't have done first.

Bottom line: Yoga is a fantastic way to enhance strength and endurance, but you need to make sure that you have a good teacher who will help you achieve your goals and will not put your aging body at risk for injury.

What is Pilates about?

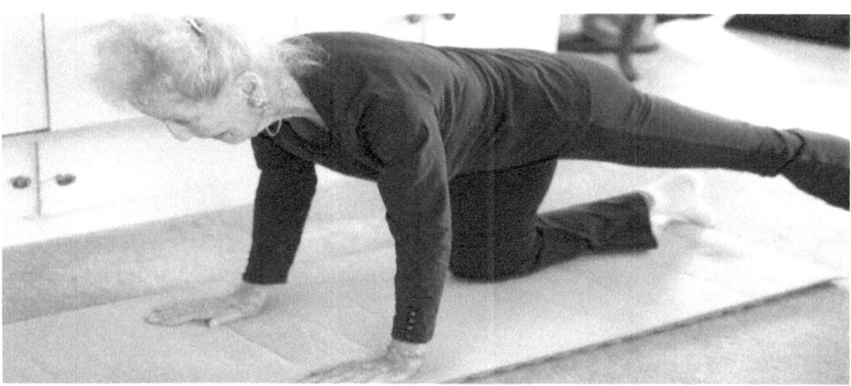

Pilates is a kind of exercise that involves a combination of floor movements and the use of specialized equipment to improve strength and flexibility. It focuses especially on strengthening the core muscles and uses dynamic and isotonic stretches along with different exercises.

What are Pilates Advantages?

Pilates is good for the aging body because it strengthens the muscles, particularly the core that leads to better posture, improves balance, and increases flexibility and motion range. It can also be better for beginners, and can easily be adapted to help target specific injuries for recovery.

What are Pilates' Disadvantages?

Some of Pilates' drawbacks are that they won't help with weight loss, the exercises take a lot of effort to perform correctly, progress is difficult to track which makes it difficult to know how far you have come, and if you have a specific problem, it can be difficult to get the individual attention you need in a classroom environment.

Bottom Line: Pilates can be a great way to become more flexible and to increase your physical strength, but it may be difficult for people with physical limitations to find an ideal setting where their concerns can be addressed properly.

Last Word: Both yoga and Pilates can be useful as an aging body stretch training program, but not every person can step into both yoga or pilates class, so take your time and find the right one for you if you want to follow one of those routes.

Chapter 6 – Common Stumbling Blocks to Stretch Training & Dangers to be Aware Of

There are a number of stumbling blocks that can keep people from stretch training as well as a few dangers that you need to be aware of before you begin. First, we'll look at some of the things that might keep you from doing stretch training and show you a few simple ways to overcome it.

Lack of Time

Many people feel that they simply don't have time to do stretch workouts because it does take a while to make sure all of your muscles have been properly stretched. However, if you look at your schedule more closely, you might find some huge chunks of time while watching TV. Combine this time with your stretch training and you won't get bored during the stretching and can use your TV time wisely.

Movement is painful

It can be hard to want your muscles to stretch and move your joints when they hurt, so bear in mind that what you're doing will help eliminate this pain over time. Also, most stretches can be modified so that they are not painful but are still effective. Be sure not to overdo it when starting first. Take things slowly, and move your own pace forward.

Lack of Energy

We fully understand that your aging body has less energy than it used to have, but don't let that stop you from doing what's best for your body. Stretch training on your body is easy and can actually make you feel more energized as it improves the circulation of your blood which can help you feel more alert and awake.

Now, let's look at some of the dangers you need to be aware of in stretch training.

Not Warming Up

 Imagine your muscles like rubber bands. If you're trying to stretch them when they're cold, they'll probably tear or even snap in two. But if you warm them up first, then they're going to be able to stretch farther and won't break. In the same way, if you move straight into passive or isotopic stretches without warming your muscles up first, you might easily hurt your muscles.

Improper Stretches

If you turn your limb the wrong way during stretch training, you may place too much pressure on the joint or the muscle which can lead to an injury. That is why it's better for someone who has never regularly done stretch training to find a trainer or instructor who can help them learn the correct way to stretch in order to prevent that risk.

Falling

This is a common problem with the aging body because falls become more dangerous and more likely as the balance will become weakened with age. While this is a potential danger during stretch training because certain stretches do need balance, there are plenty of things that you can do to reduce this risk such as using a wall or sturdy chair for support or practicing with a strong partner who can aid you.

Chapter 7 – Overview of Stretch Workouts for Beginners

We will give you an overview of a stretch workout in this part of the course which has two basic parts: the warm-up and the stretching. While most workouts require a cool-down phase after the main part of your workout, you can skip that with stretch training, as it doesn't require your muscles to work hard enough to cool down afterward.

Warm-up

As mentioned in the last segment, stretching your muscles without first warming up can lead to muscle tears and injuries, which is why it's so important to have your body ready for at least 10 minutes of stretch. Fortunately, warm-up is very easy and physical exercise is also helpful in boosting muscle strength and circulation.

The quickest warm-up for a stretch routine is to walk for 10 minutes. If you're doing your stretch training at home, you can walk up and down the hallway, or even walk in the room. Since you're going to stretch your arm muscles as well, it's necessary to move your arms more than you usually would while walking, almost as if you were running quickly.

Stretch Workout

During your stretch workout, you'll need to work through all the big muscle groups to ensure you cover all of them. The 11 main muscle groups to be analyzed include forearms, biceps , triceps, shoulders, trapezoids, chest, belly, back, quadriceps , hamstrings, and calves. If you use our stretch routine from the next section or make your own, make sure you 're covering all of the major muscle groups.

You need to use a variety of stretch types too. Dynamic and active stretches are perfect for muscle strength development when relaxing, which is also good for bone mass enhancement, so if you're concerned about bone loss, you might want to try these. Passive and isotopic stretches are much easier to do, making them ideal for people interested in balancing out.

Make sure every stretch for the amount of time specified for that stretch is complete. There's a reason you 're supposed to do that long-term, and why it probably won't hurt to do it for longer, if you do it for a shorter period of time it won't be nearly as successful as that means you won't get the results you 're after.

Another thing to keep in mind during stretch workout is that stretching shouldn't be painful. You may feel the muscle stretching and may experience some slight discomfort, but if you feel pain in your muscles, this is a sign that you are either doing the stretching poorly or pushing yourself too hard, too fast, and you need to work your way up to stretching that far.

When to Cool Down

You will benefit from a mild cool down if you want to do dynamic stretching. This can consist of just walking for 10 minutes and/or doing a few passive or isotopic stretches to help your muscles relax fully after your stretching routine.

Chapter 8 – Sample Stretch Workouts

Within this segment, we'll provide you with a list of the best stretches for each of the 11 muscle groups. You can use these for your stretch exercise, or you can find ones that are better for every group of muscles to do. Always warm-up for a minimum of 10 minutes before you start so your muscles is ready to stretch. You do want to make sure you keep for 30 seconds to 1 minute each period.

Forearm – Standing extensor stretch, standing wrist flexor stretch, assisted forearm stretch, and wrist spins are the best stretches for the forearm.

Biceps – You'll want to try the standing biceps stretch, biceps wall stretch, wrist-rotation biceps stretch, door biceps stretch and seated bent-knee biceps stretch with your biceps.

Triceps - Use the overhead triceps stretch and cross-body triceps stretch to stretch the triceps.

Shoulder – You'll want to do chin retractions, neck rolls, shoulder raises, shoulder rotate and the standing wall stretch to boost your shoulder flexibility.

Trapeziums – The best stretches for losing muscles of your trapeziums are the stretch of forwarding trapeziums, the stretch of side trapeziums, and stretch of diagonal trapezia.

Chest – You'll need to stretch the wall, elbow wrap stretch, backbend stretch, lying chest stretch, and standing chest extension to extend your chest.

Abdominal-You want to do the lying abdominal stretch, standing abdominal stretch, and abdominal rotations with the abdominal muscles.

Back – You'll want to try stretching the knee to the chest, lying knee twist, performs seated stretch and yoga poses like cobra, restful post and cat/cow poses to stretch your back muscles.

Quadriceps – There are three stretches perfect for quadriceps: the stretch of kneeling quadriceps, the stretch of standing quadriceps, and the stretch of field quadriceps.

Hamstrings-The hamstring roller, hamstring twist, adapted hamstring twist, butterfly, open-air stretch, and single-leg loop are some of the better stretches for the hamstrings.

Calves – Standing calf stretch, wall calf stretch, and downward dog yoga pose are the perfect exercises for the calves.

Aiming for Muscle Classes

Then you may need to do multiple sets of stretches for certain muscles to address different muscle groups that are especially stiff or sore. You can also recommend keeping each stretch for up to 3 minutes each to allow room to spread out more of your muscle fibers inside that muscle. You should also do these stretching exercises about once a day to help further develop flexibility.

Targeting Joints

If you have a specific joint in which you want to increase your range of motion, then you need to focus on the muscle groups that control the joint. Think about what muscles are on either side of the joint, then do further muscle stretches. If your knees are a problem, for example, then you'll want to stretch your quadriceps, hamstrings, and calves more than other muscles.

Chapter 9 - Tools/Resources/Apps to Help with Staying Limber into Older Age

If you think it would be difficult to remain limber at an older age then make sure to use these devices, resources, and features to help you achieve your stability goals. Be sure to use the resources that are most appropriate for you personally when it comes to stretching training, as not every single resource is best for every person.

Foam Roller

A foam roller is one of the best devices you can purchase and will help you with your stretch training. Since it is so powerful, it can be painful too, particularly when you use it first. However, this is a great tool to have if you want good results, particularly in your back and calves. You will need to hire a personal trainer or attend a foam roller class to learn properly how to use one, and the type that is right for you.

Lacrosse Ball

A lacrosse ball is another useful tool you could consider buying. These provide you with a way to do self-massage in places where you need some extra support, such as the neck or back. A lacrosse ball helps you to place pressure at a certain point where you can have knots of connective tissues. Removal of these knotted fibers will help you feel better and quickly become more mobile.

Rope

We have mentioned using stretch bands before which some give in them, but you can also use a simple piece of rope or even a towel to help make isotopic stretches resistant. Using a couple of ropes or towels of different lengths can help you improve stretch performance.

Classes

You can take many different classes which can help by being a local community of like-minded people and by getting a trained teacher to show you how to stretch correctly, without hurting yourself. Take the time to find a class that's right for you, and don't be afraid to ask if you can take one class to test it out before you commit to more.

Personal Trainer / Physical Therapist

When you have a specific health issue that needs attention, you will need to opt to work one-on-one with a personal trainer or physical therapist who will make sure that the workouts you're doing can actually help you better rather than making it worse. A good physical therapist can usually be recommended by your doctor and many gyms have personal trainers that can help.

Applications

Another perfect way to help you stick to your stretch routine is by phone applications. Some exercise apps will also allow you to build your own exercise plan where you can add stretches and decide how long each of them you want to do, then let them play. Then when you're ready to stretch, all you need to do is start the workout and follow the directions along with.

Using a combination of these tools helps you to keep track of your stretch training plan and be successful. We'll give you even more ideas in the next section that you can use to make stretching out part of your daily routine.

Conclusion – Tips to Add Stretching into Your Daily Life Long-term

Congratulations on making this short, introductory report about basic secrets to remain limber and healthy as a senior until the end.

You may be shocked to learn the majority of people who start something never completes it.

Take the time to make progress at your own pace. This isn't a race. The more you understand and understand what happens when you take a stretching & stability course the better the performance.

If you really want to succeed, then considering long-term planning, everything you do for your body must be in mind. Such adjustments you make and the diet that you adopt is not supposed to be temporary. They're supposed to be part of a healthier lifestyle you're adopting to hold off the weight you've gained and helped you keep yourself safe.

Equally important as doing the stretches properly is doing them every day, that's why we're going to give you some tips in this section that you can use to add stretching into your everyday life so you can stick with it and continue to reap the benefits of a stretch training program.

Set timetable

You want to determine exactly when you are going to do that before you start your stretch training program. You may want to do your stretching first thing in the morning if you're afraid you'll get too busy during the day and forget about that. If you know that you're going to have better luck after lunch or right before bed, then prepare to devote the time to stretch out preparation and not let anything else mess with it.

Using Friends and Family

Easily use the people around you is one of the easiest ways to help keep you on board with your stretch work. If you can find a stretching buddy, spending time together, and keeping each other accountable can be a nice way to make sure that you stretch as much as you can. It might even be easier to do these stretches with someone else to assist you.

Doing easy things like sharing on Facebook about your workout is another way your family and friends can get great support. If you undertake to write about your workout every day

Alternatively, let one person know when you're finishing your stretch workout, then you can remain accountable and get a ton of encouragement to keep you going.

Join a Community Online

You can join tons of online communities which will help you stay on track with your stretch training. These are both great sites for asking questions about what you are doing and getting tips about how to get the most out of your stretch training. If you're looking to join a good online community, be sure to look at how active and helpful the members are.

Create a Calendar

Using a calendar that you mark on the days you've finished your stretch training is a good way to note that you need to do it every day, and a good way to be accountable. When you're done for the day, you can mark days clearly by putting a big happy face on the calendar, or have fun with it by buying colorful stickers to mark the days.

Recompense yourself

It's a smart way to use quick constructive reinforcement to keep yourself on track. It could be that at the end of each training session you give yourself a small healthy treat, or that you allow yourself to buy something special at the end of a week that you went to training every day. Make sure anything you choose as your reward is something that will not hurt your health.

By prioritizing stretch training, you'll see the positive results you 're looking for

Bonus Chapter – Advanced Stretch Workouts

You'll want to start moving on to more advanced stretch exercises once you've learned the basics of the passive stretches that we mentioned earlier. Advanced stretch workouts will allow you to go beyond where you're now and help you strive to be even more versatile. Make sure you slowly add advanced stretches to your routine so you don't get yourself injured.

Yoga Poses

There are a variety of yoga poses that can only be performed by someone who has mastered the fundamentals of stretching altogether. If you take yoga classes as your main type of stretch training, you should always start with a beginner class or one specifically tailored for an aging body. When you're ready to try out a more advanced class, your instructor will tell you.

Pilates

Because in addition to stretches, Pilates involves a number of movements, it is not for everyone, but it is great for building muscle strength along with flexibility. Many moves by Pilates can be done at home with nothing but a yoga mat, but many others require specialized equipment. Fortunately, Pilates classes can be found which have what you need: special equipment and trained instructors.

Active Stretching

You'll want to add aggressive stretching to your arsenal, rather than just passive stretching. These stretches are much harder because you need to use the muscle to keep the limb in place. This, alongside versatility, makes them perfect for building energy. Since successful stretching is using the muscles, after a stretching session you'll probably need to cool down with some light walking.

Dynamic Stretching

If you have balance problems, be very careful when doing dynamic stretching, because it involves a lot of movement, usually one leg at a time. Although you can use a wall or a solid chair for support, these can be challenging for people with issues with balance. If you can add these to your routine, however, dynamic stretches are great to at the same time boost flexibility and muscle strength.

Using Resources

Throughout the course, we have listed a few basic tools you can use to enhance your stretch training. We've addressed stretch or resistance bands, incline boards, yoga mats, stretch machines, foam rollers, lacrosse balls, and a rope or towel to study. All these things are intended to help you stretch out better.

You'll probably only want to add one or two of these things at a time, so look at each stretch training tool to see what works best for you to tackle specific problems or

Muscle bands. Then, once you have mastered using one tool, you can add another to it until you have what you need for your stretch training needs.

Thanks for taking the time to read this course on aging body stretching. We hope we have given you all the knowledge you need to be able to stay limber even as time appears to work against you. You can keep your muscles and joints limber no matter how old you are by being patient and using all of your resources wisely.

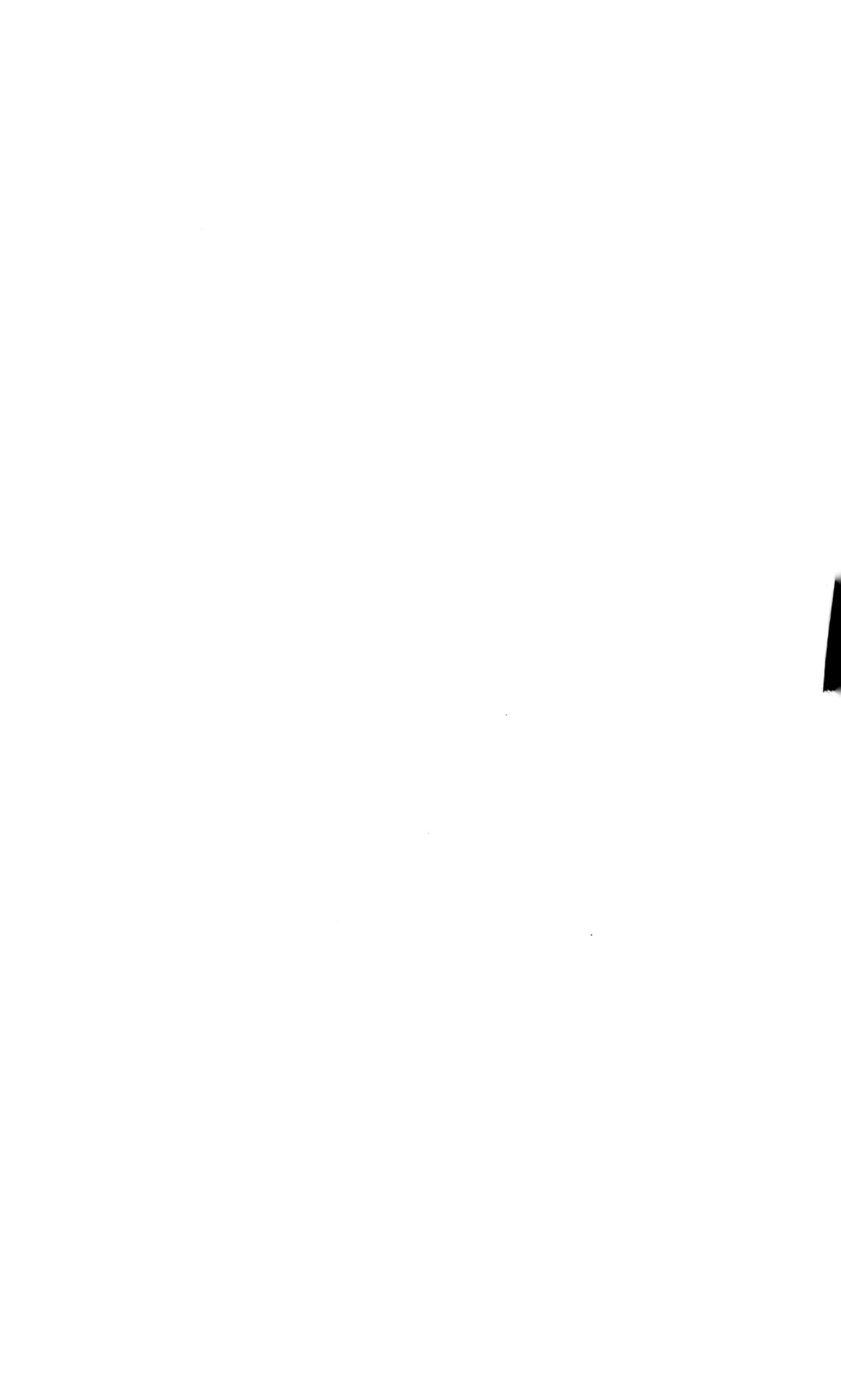

www.ingramcontent.com/pod-product-compliance
Lightning Source LLC
Chambersburg PA
CBHW020946160726
47993CB00007B/2960